T0156692

DIABETES
ANNIHILATED—NATURALLY
MY STARTLING AND ADVENTUROUS DRUG-FREE REVERSAL OF DIABETES

M. DALE CAMPBELL

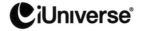

DIABETES ANNIHILATED—NATURALLY
MY STARTLING AND ADVENTUROUS
DRUG-FREE REVERSAL OF DIABETES

iUniverse books may be ordered through booksellers or by contacting:

iUniverse
1663 Liberty Drive
Bloomington, IN 47403
www.iuniverse.com
1-800-Authors (1-800-288-4677)

ISBN: 978-1-4917-9060-1 (sc)
ISBN: 978-1-4917-9059-5 (hc)
ISBN: 978-1-4917-9063-2 (e)

Library of Congress Control Number: 2016903073

Print information available on the last page.

iUniverse rev. date: 06/09/2016

CONTENTS

INTRODUCTION, RATIONALE, AND ACKNOWLEDGMENTS

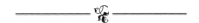

My doctor lied to me about my diabetes—not intentionally or maliciously, of course. Dr. Amin has been our trusted family physician for more than thirty years and has taken great care of each of us under varying health challenges with loving, professional care. But when he said I would "never control my blood glucose without" the drug he prescribed, I took it as a challenge. I went straight home, bypassing all the pharmacies on the way, and cured myself—naturally.

How can I say that I am cured? Dr. Amin said, "You should write a book so I can tell my other diabetic patients about your story." So here it is, Dr. Amin. Also, I write this for anyone who is concerned about pre-diabetes or diabetes. This is just my story, and I make no claims about your success. However, a number of friends have succeeded in duplicating my story in their own ways.

I have heard one natural doctor—among many other skeptics—say that diabetes can never be cured, just controlled. However, after four years, my blood sugar rises and falls just as nature planned it—even with sweet things.

I also have an amazing A1C ranging between 5.6 and 5.8—down from 12.1 when diagnosed—all without drugs.

I typically awaken with fasting glucose levels ranging from 70 to 88 mg/dl. After a meal, my level rises to between 130 mg/dl and 150 mg/dl, which is well below the 398 mg/dl when I was diagnosed.

I believe you can do it too—naturally. Read on. You'll see.

Writing this book is the result of the persistent encouragement of my MME (Master Minds of Excellence) team. Renee, Sandy, and Margaret function as my personal board of directors—along with many others who realize that my experience may also inspire the millions of type 2 diabetics in the United States and around the world.

Though I still monitor my blood sugar, after just eighteen months of an incredibly fun roller-coaster ride, I can safely say that this is the time to write this work. I am cured. My diabetes has been reversed.

My children, Alex and Brittanie, may need this someday, and I write this for them, but I especially dedicate this to my grandson, Dante, who is almost two years old at the time of the initial writing. This is one of the many stories that he can tell about his "Appa." I hope he learns quickly to live according to the knowledge of the connection between making healthy choices, glorifying God, and experiencing a better quality of life.

A special thanks goes to my wife, Fuchsia; my daughter, Brittanie; my son, Mike; and my daughter-in-law, Valerie, for putting up with all the "aromatic" experiments at making healthy, delicious, interesting meals in the kitchen at odd times day and night each week. I also wish to thank all my friends—in particular, Jackie, Meredith, Reggie, and Garth (my favorite chiropractor and also a high school and university classmate)—who supported me in my quest for natural healing and reversal of this rather insidious disease.

I hope this will lead my family, friends, and others to healthier living as God intended. I also hope it leads to accelerated success for all those burdened with the challenges of type 2 diabetes—not in controlling it but in *curing* it.

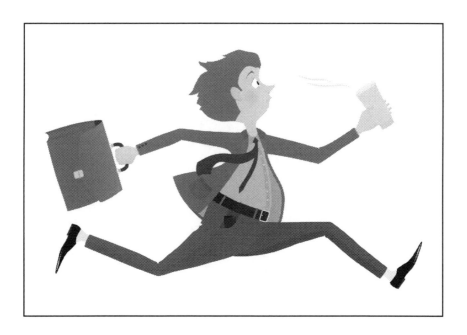

Chapter 1

THE JOURNEY BEGINS

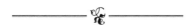

It is early on a Sunday morning in April 2011 as I start to write this story for you. The previous evening, we had dinner with some friends to celebrate a birthday in the group. I went light with dinner and had a delicious roasted-vegetable sandwich, fries, ketchup, hot sauce, and some water. It was really not so bad, but I did top it all off with a huge portion of a rather sweet and flavorful bread pudding.

After returning from the restaurant, we went immediately to prepare for bed and get some sleep. I checked my blood sugar just before crawling in, and it was at a healthy 159 mg/dl, still within an hour after downing all that sugar. Upon rising this morning, the reading is an exciting 98 mg/dl.

My story does not start there. I must take you back about two years earlier—just a little before my grandson was born.

In June 2009, I decided on a whim to see my doctor for a checkup. It was almost three years since I had seen any doctor, and past the age of fifty, that's not a good practice. When Dr. Amin. asked me why I came to see him, I said, "I have a little time on my hands and thought I should stop in to verify how healthy I am." My cocky response tells you my state of mind. I was feeling great. I had lots of energy and enthusiasm. I was highly productive in my career as a traveling educational consultant and actively involved in weekend and evening activities.

I had good reason, beyond just feeling great, to expect an excellent report from Dr. Amin. I always thought I was the healthiest guy anywhere.

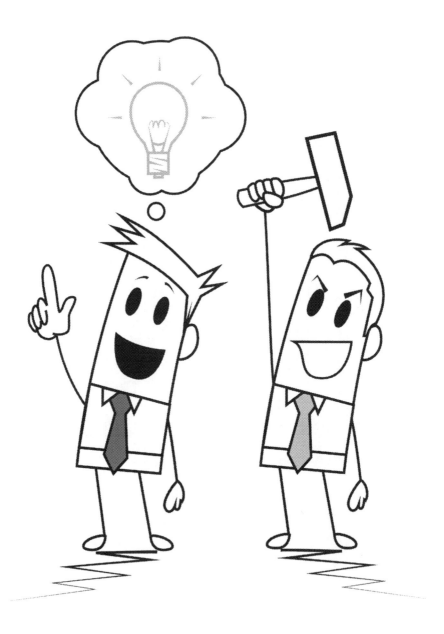

Chapter 2

STRANGE ENCOUNTERS AND A FEW GOOD, BAD HABITS

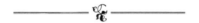

Why would I think I was so healthy? My first life-changing experience with natural healing occurred in 1977. A patch of hair just behind my right ear fell out within weeks of our wedding. (I really wanted to blame my new bride for this, but I found no basis to do so.) Many doctors named my condition alopecia, but they provided no solution to restore my hair.

About three months later, some friends introduced us to Dr. Curtis Golden, ND (naturopathic physician). I began to understand the power of diet, homeopathy, acupuncture, acupressure, herbs, and zone therapy with low-level electromagnetic fields to heal the body. My hair grew back in a few short weeks after eating raw nuts, seeds, and grains. A little manipulation to my cervical vertebrae improved blood flow through my neck. I was hooked on natural remedies from that time. (See more about this in chapter 11.)

Later, I studied acupuncture, Jin Shin Do, Jin Jin Jit Su, and other touch therapies with Dr. Paul Zmiewski and Dr. Brian Manuele at the Midwest Center for Oriental Medicine in Chicago.

Additionally, I ate rather healthily: no pop (soda), very little red meat, lots of vegetables, and juices. I refused—and still refuse—to purchase any item with additives, coloring, manufactured flavors, or preservatives. I avoided every beverage with added sugar, and I limited refined sugars. I enjoyed a relatively low-carb, high-protein, and vegetable diet for about ten years except for occasional pastries and ice cream. I also included many organic foods, vitamins, and mineral supplements. What could have happened to me?

When I completed my checkup and tests, I was totally stunned to hear Dr. Amin say, "You have diabetes. Come into my office right away." After his compelling tirade, a review of my data, and a prescription for Metformin, I still denied the possibility. I went out to consume my favorite banana split combination at Plush Horse, the best ice cream I have found in my entire state. After all, how could diabetes happen to the healthiest guy in town? I was definitely in denial. With a background like mine, wouldn't you be in denial too?

However, like most of us, I relished sweet things and had a little health game going. This is where good habits can turn out to be bad habits. I would only have sweet things without preservatives. Better yet, I would choose cookies and pastries with organic ingredients, and I only consumed 100 percent natural juices. My diet was really better than average, but it was not really great (as I can now attest).

Natural fruit juices—even straight from the fruit—are really not natural in the strictest sense. Dr. Ellecom, a clinical psychologist and friend, explained recently how one glass of orange juice can equal as many as six oranges. The sugar impact to the body is likely much more intense and rapid than God intended. Eating six oranges would likely take more time and would also contain more of the natural enzymes and fiber to help the body process it.

This, I believe, was my downfall. I had too much of a good thing—natural fruit juices in huge quantities almost every day for more than twenty years. I would consume up to a gallon of orange juice on a hot summer Sunday. I avoided water like the plague, and when I traveled for work, I constantly consumed 100 percent natural, no-sugar-added juices from vending machines, food marts, health-food stores, and airport cafés. I would even leave without a purchase if they did not have this quality available.

If you are concerned about diabetes in your life, check where you may be abusing your body with too many sweets. Consider where you may consume high levels of non-sweet carbohydrates, such as pasta, rice, potatoes, or fried dumplings. According to Obi Obadike, world-renown fitness trainer and nutrition consultant, research shows that most adults in a sedentary lifestyle should not have as many carbs as we all tend to consume. He himself has linked to a feature of 40 low-carb foods that help reduce the waistline at http://www.bodybuilding.com/fun/bbmainnut.htm.[16] The next chapter makes the case for this understanding and analysis regarding carbohydrates.

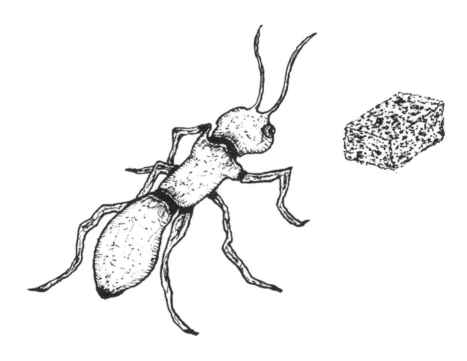

Chapter 3

Possible Causes, Symptoms, and the Ant Test for Diabetes

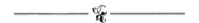

Of the possible causes of adult-onset or type 2 diabetes, lifestyle is perhaps the most significant. This includes nutrition, exercise, and proper rest. Even a healthy diet with good sweets (juices, granola with honey, etc.) in excess can cause the blood to maintain high levels of glucose. Cells in the body can begin to resist the insulin transport of glucose across the cell membrane. For people who are overweight and have poor muscle tone, the diminished muscular demand for glucose is compounded by the fact that the fat molecules tend to block the entry of glucose through the cell membrane. Their blood glucose levels remain constantly high.

Another key cause of diabetes is reduced insulin production in the pancreas—Islets of Langerhans—which acupuncture and dietary regimens can correct in many cases. Dr. Gabriel Cousens and Dr. Neal Barnard found one patient with type 1 diabetes who was fully cured with a vegan diet along with many other type 2 diabetics. Since reduced insulin production was not my experience, the information presented here relates to the more common type 2 diabetes where there is cell membrane resistance to insulin.

I grew up in a third-world country where I overheard adults describing a very interesting test for diabetes: Put some of your urine where ants can easily find it. If they gather around it, your blood sugar is likely high.

It is amazing that folklore and modern medicine agree here. Glucosuria describes a condition where the kidneys are not able to reabsorb the sugar from the fluids that will later become urine. This is most often due to high concentrations of sugar in the bloodstream (diabetes) and the resulting high sugar concentration in the fluids of the kidney, which is too much for the kidneys to reabsorb. A urine dipstick at home or a lab test can quickly tell if there is sugar in the urine. Feel free to use the official ant test for glucosuria and see what happens.

What other indicators accompany symptoms of diabetes besides ants? Sugar in the urine is often accompanied by fatigue, unexplained weight loss, excessive thirst or hunger, and frequent urination.

I ignored all of these key symptoms—especially frequent urination and moderate weight loss—for quite a while. First, I was really glad for the weight loss and thought that it came from exercising and watching my food intake.

Be careful to look out for these indicators because I ignored the frequent urination. I thought it would go away. I had to urinate between and during meetings, on the highway, and on airplanes. I went up to three times per night—whether I was at home or in a hotel.

In fact, as a workshop leader, my audiences got frequent breaks because of my need to use the bathroom. Additionally, I had bouts of dizziness and an inability to think clearly, even during my presentations.

About four years prior to my diagnosis, after a vigorous and enthusiastic start to a workshop in rural Kentucky, I felt a little chest pain and dizziness. I noticed that my speech was slurred. Some of the participants took me to the hospital, but the tests found nothing. I was kept overnight for observation and discharged in the morning with no indications of anything being wrong.

What did I have for breakfast just minutes before the event? Three or four glasses of 100 percent pure orange juice, scrambled eggs, toast, and two Danish pastries. It was not my usual breakfast, but at the hotel, it was the quick breakfast route. I was running just a bit late. I downed the breakfast that was there. I suspect that my body was beginning to develop insulin resistance. I had many instances of this feeling—not quite as intense—typically after a breakfast with lots of juice. I discovered that if I just kept lecturing and presenting, the feeling would go away. With just a few changes in lifestyle, I no longer have any of these symptoms.

Please pay close attention to the messages from your body. I am actually quite fortunate not to have experienced significant tissue damage or worse.

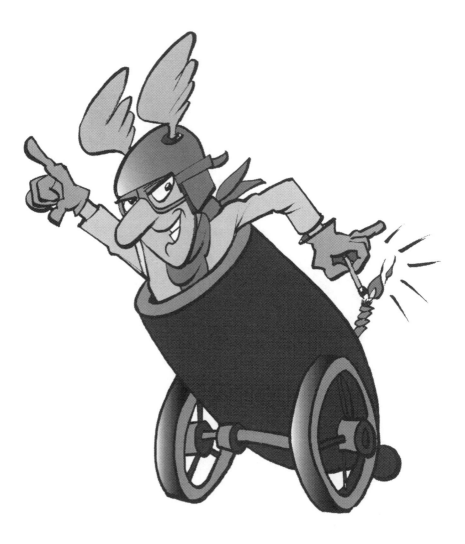

Chapter 4

DANGERS OF DIABETES I CARELESSLY MISSED

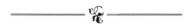

Persistently high blood sugar levels lead to a tremendous amount of cellular and tissue damage over time. Wounds tend not to heal, eyesight diminishes, and cellular fluid balance is turned upside down, causing frequent urination. The Chinese describe diabetes as a wasting away of muscle tissue which results in rapid weight loss in some cases.

Additionally, nerve damage looms large on the list of dangers. Diminished eyesight makes this evident. I went to my optometrist to get new glasses. I went back to him eight weeks later to have him correct the prescription for my glasses. I did not realize the possibility of nerve damage in the retina. This condition is known as diabetic retinopathy. The feeling of diminished eyesight is very strange. I could see absolutely fine to read and drive, but there was a kind of emptiness in the images. I felt the need to refocus more frequently in order to see the outer edges of an object, especially distant ones.

I know I frustrated the optometrist. He reviewed and retested everything, and I had the perfect prescription. A year later, I was diagnosed with the disease. I carried on with life, and some days were better than others. I had a good vision on some days and poor vision on other days. I was just too busy with life to take care of life. Shame on me! After all, I was Mr. Healthy and did not care to make the connection.

Please don't take chances with your health. You may not be as lucky as I have been. I no longer have these issues, and my eyesight has been restored.

Eyesight was not the only factor, however. I also ignored my tingling feet for quite a while. When Dr. Amin went through his soft-spoken, firm, almost angry tirade about the dangers of diabetes and the immediate care needed, he asked me about my feet. I remembered the sensations in my feet that went back almost two years.

I was in a sales position at the time. I found that if I hired a driver, I could increase my efficiency and turnaround for proposals. I was able to use the driving time for creative solutions to challenges and to do Internet research on the way from one customer to another. I began having tingles in my feet, which was the beginning of diabetic neuropathy. I had no idea what was going on, but I assumed that the Midwest winters were getting to me as I got older. I eventually got to the point where the feeling didn't bother me much, and life continued in oblivion. Please do not ignore symptoms of any kind. Check them out immediately.

In developed countries with great medical care, the causes of many symptoms cannot be identified, especially with traditional allopathic medicine. Do not let that stop you. Go to an MD, DC, ND, PhD, or L. Acu, to learn what is going on with your body. They don't have the complete picture all the time, but if you are armed with information from a variety of sources and medical perspectives, you can usually make more intelligent decisions about your care.

With neuropathy of the feet, the key danger occurs when you get cut and feel nothing. It festers and can potentially become serious. The nerve endings no longer communicate to the brain. Many diabetics get infections from nicks while cutting their toenails because they do not even feel it. The cuts go unnoticed, and infections set in. This is another danger, but there is more.

I had friends in my home who were visiting from Florida. The gentleman was on his way to a funeral. His brother-in-law had also passed away recently. Diabetes caused both premature deaths. One of them was a physician who ignored the required lifestyle changes and had two legs amputated prior to his premature death. Get regular checkups and adjust your lifestyle to ensure optimum health.

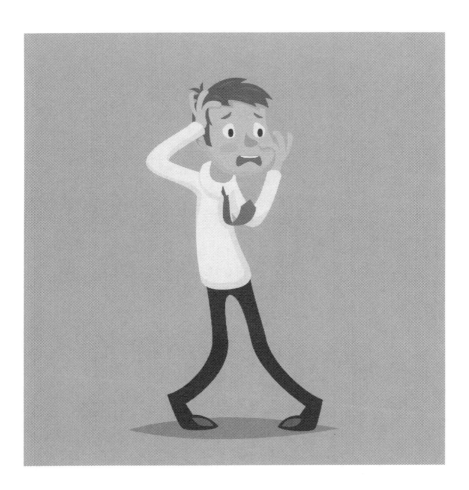

Chapter 5

THE SCARE: "I MAY NOT BE CONSCIOUS" – MY DOCTOR'S UNWITTING CHALLENGE

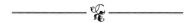

After my splurge at Plush Horse, I stashed the prescription from Dr. Amin in a drawer and vowed to find another way. By telling me the truth about Metformin, Dr. Amin scared me. He'd obviously rehearsed the precautionary statements and disclaimers before that day. In the case of an emergency room visit, he said, "You should inform the emergency room staff about your use of Metformin to avoid any possible complications with emergency room care."

What if I'm not conscious when I go to the emergency room? That scared me.

As I drove home after my third visit with Dr. Amin, I reflected on my previous experiences with natural healing and his unwitting challenge. He challenged me by saying, "You will not be able to control your sugar without drugs. You have to enjoy yourself too."

I took that to mean that I should take the drug and eat and drink whatever I wanted. That was the giveaway. What a novel idea! Diabetes could be controlled by diet and without drugs! A surge of energy kicked me into full gear, and I set out on a path to take control of my health via natural means—without pharmaceutical drugs.

Fortunately, it was the beginning of summer, and I worked mostly from home. My schedule was mostly based on discretionary time. I was convinced that more than 90 percent of diseases and adverse health conditions have natural remedies. I immediately set out on a path of discovery. I typed "cure diabetes naturally" in my Google search. I wanted direct answers, a clear, accurate understanding of this disease, and a way to get rid of it without drugs. After about an hour of searching through meaningless leads and information, the search yielded a book for sale from Barton Publishers. *The Diabetes Reversal Report* was priced as an impulse buy for people who really wanted to know about curing diabetes.[3] The title got my attention. I immediately downloaded the book, and what I learned from it and numerous other sources was the basis for my incredible journey to cure myself of diabetes.

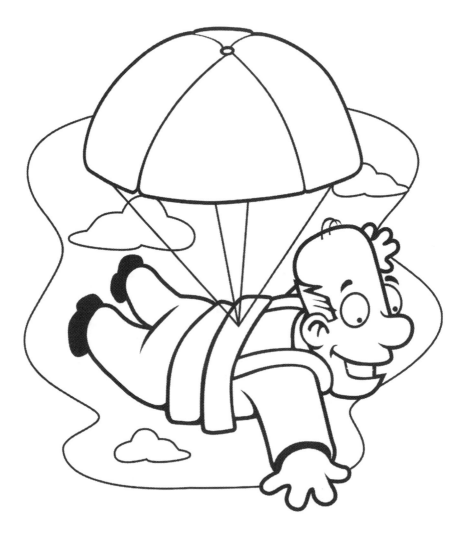

Chapter 6

THE FIVE ESSENTIAL INGREDIENTS FOR SUCCESS

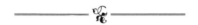

There are five essential ingredients for my success. My success is the result of much more than the information contained in my research. It has much to do with my core values and my beliefs. Our beliefs determine our values, our values lead us to action, and our actions lead us to outcomes.

Ingredient #1—Tweaking My Core Values and Worldview

If we really want to bring lasting change to any aspect of life, we must first clearly identify with or change the relevant belief system from which we operate our lives. In this case, we must identify with or develop a value system that makes health and fitness or freedom from illness or disease a part of the core. If relevant core values and their supporting beliefs are not present, you will not likely succeed in this or any other serious endeavor.

I hasten to tell you that this road requires discipline and commitment. The joy of it must be in the doing of it for the sole reason that doing so makes us congruent with our core values, which makes all of this really fun.

For a more in-depth discourse on core values for all of life's challenges, please e-mail me at TheSmarterVision@gmail.com. You will learn how to create and live by your core values for the most complete sense of joy, satisfaction, and fulfillment in life. In the meantime, let's deal with the topic of diabetes.

Ingredient #2—Confidence in Natural Healing

Think about your beliefs regarding natural healing, fitness, lifestyle changes, self-analysis, and setting goals. Are you determined to be healthy—naturally? Really? If the answer is a resounding yes, then success will come with minimal challenge and effort. If your answer is anything less than that, you can make it, but the struggles and challenges will be proportionate to your lack of passion for good health the natural way.

Ingredient #3—Take Full Responsibility for Your Health

This ingredient is about a change in role. You must accept responsibility for your health. Many of us go to the doctor for him/her to make us better. This is a fair expectation in many cases. However, in the search for answers, it became very clear that most medical doctors have no real knowledge of natural health concepts due to the type of training they experience. Therefore, your new role can include health researcher, scientist, physician, consultant, and any other role you need to make this happen for you. The fun is in the trying—and ultimately in the winning. If you want to go straight to the win, stop reading right now. Learning, understanding, and participating willingly in the process create the win.

Ingredient #4—Dare to Win the Game of Hurdles

The fun is in the trying. I made the commitment to cure my diabetes even with my travels. My bigger challenge—after preparing my meals, packing them in insulated containers, and making reservations only in hotels with refrigerators—was the TSA. Airport security was high everywhere.

Here's what I think I looked like to the TSA: strange bag, lots of strange items—some of them liquids—and electronics for my job (speakers, microphones, and lots of wires).

Just about every pass through security yielded a familiar sound: "Bag check!" I felt the pressure of holding up the lines of other hurried travelers. I even missed a few flights as a result of my routine. I eventually learned how to cook a little drier and package some items with checked luggage—especially my alkaline water bottles. My boss at the time even questioned my water bottles on my expense report.

Another incident occurred in the remote town of O'Neill, Nebraska. I spent one night there in utter confusion. I had forgotten my glucometer on the plane and had nothing to measure my blood sugar. My heart was racing, and I could not sleep. I was not sure why any of it was occurring. Since it was a small town, no pharmacies were open for fifty miles. The only hospital in town informed me that I would need to make an emergency room visit to get my blood sugar checked. I said, "That's a very expensive glucose check."

I did not want the medical label on my record anywhere else. At my doctor was bad enough. I prayed for wisdom and prepared for a rough night. I alerted the hotel attendant that I was not feeling well and asked him to check on me every thirty minutes or so. He agreed.

During the wee hours of the morning, in my little arsenal of health products, I found a mineral powder from www.claydoc.com, which I affectionately called mud. I had not so far observed any impact of this powder on my diabetes, but the properties for health restoration were supposed to be amazing. At about two o'clock, I prepared the mixture with my alkaline water and gulped it down after letting it sit for about two hours—per the instructions. In about fifteen minutes, my racing heart quieted down, and I was able to get a few minutes of sleep before rising at five thirty to get ready for the day. That experience was scary and appears to have been a psychosomatic reaction to having no glucometer. In any case, I had something natural that worked great and got me a little sleep.

Ingredient #5—Do Your Own Research

Another benefit of this experience was learning to follow a routine. Dr. Yurasek, PhD in acupuncture and now a good friend, identified that the best way to learn about the body is to have a routine or to try different routines over time. Check your blood sugar every day at the same time and eat at the same times every day. Try different schedules to see what works best. This makes it easier to compare the data and make observations about the body's response to your daily cycle and food intake. This was very challenging when traveling, but I did it with few exceptions.

I found ways to check blood sugar without being noticed in airplanes, conference rooms, and bathrooms. If it was time to eat or check blood sugar, I excused myself and followed the regimen. Ultimately, this helped me understand what foods affected me more than others and what time for dinner worked best to get a good fasting blood glucose in the mornings. Not eating after five thirty in the evening allowed me to see significant drops in blood sugar each morning. I was thrilled to see my body responding favorably to the routine. I later found that exercising in the evenings yielded better fasting glucose results as well.

I survived many challenges in the quest for understanding and a cure. I encourage you and your loved ones to take the challenge because all of that is behind me. I would not trade the experience for any other. I am able to enjoy myself with cake, ice cream, and other delights—always in moderation—but without drugs, supplements, or supports.

The five essential ingredients for success include:

- adjusting core beliefs regarding natural healing and being willing to take any informed role necessary
- having confidence that you will reverse diabetes naturally

- taking full personal responsibility for your health
- daring to win the game of hurdles and making it fun
- sticking to a routine while collecting data (eating, testing, and resting at the same times each day)

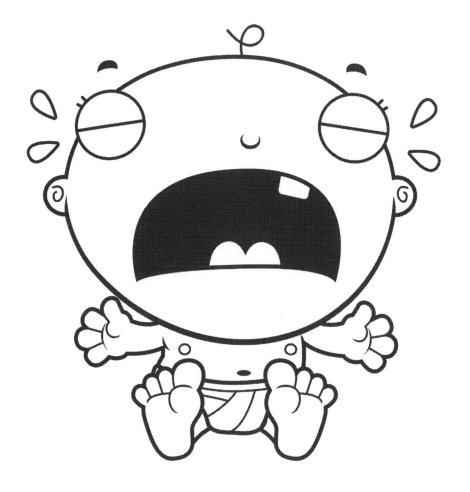

Chapter 7

SHEDDING TEARS MADE IT ALL WORTHWHILE

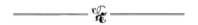

You may recall the term *homeostasis* from high school or college. Homeostasis describes a physiological process that allows an organism to maintain internal stability. In the case of diabetes, high blood sugar is a steady state the body finds "normal." One of the first things that one can change by diet is the blood sugar level. It helps the body identify with a different steady state (homeostasis).

My path to this new homeostasis started with *The Diabetes Reversal Report*. I reduced my carbohydrate intake to twenty grams per day.[3] That was about one teaspoon of brown rice, one or two slices of bread (depending on type and brand), and one or two sips of juices or sweetened beverages per day. My meals for three months consisted of organic eggs, organic chicken, organic and grass-fed beef, organic eggplant, organic tofu, and organic salad ingredients of any possible type I dared to try. I found ways to make eggplant tasty and used many vegetarian ingredients as meat substitutes. I also learned to enjoy water. With the change from juices to water, my body went into withdrawal.

I vividly recall bursting into tears at our local Trader Joe's store because I had to pass up on my favorite 100 percent juice and other healthy treats in order to stay within the twenty grams per day. I called my wife from the supermarket. Between my sobs, trembling lips, and literal tears, I wondered if I could make it. My wife convinced me that I could—and that really helped.

Sticking to twenty grams per day can be easy if you read labels carefully and count the grams in the foods you eat each day. Stay with those foods for a while. There are websites that will help you with that. Just do a web search for "carb counters" or see the "A Bibliography with Useful Resources" at the end of this book.[1]

Do not assume anything about the carbohydrate content of any food. Check it out first. For example, adzuki beans and baked beans are great sources of protein, but they are also fairly high in carbohydrates. A cooked half-cup has more than twenty-five grams of carbs. That blows your carb limit for the day. Many nuts are also high in carbs, but almonds, hazelnuts, macadamias, and others have low carbs. They are great sources of nutrition as well. If you like meat, poultry, or game (please go organic or grass-fed to minimize added hormones, drugs, and additives), you will be happy to know you can eat as much of them as you want. Most of them have zero carbs (with the exception of liver and hot dogs). This is assuming that you are preparing these items yourself and that no sauces or condiments containing sugars are being added to the recipes.

The bottom line on these lifestyle changes is that we should eat more like the original diet of humans. After creation, people's diets consisted of unprocessed foods. They were right from the ground, the tree, or the sky. The water had no added chlorine or fluoride, the vegetables had no pesticides, and the meats had no added hormones. Animals ate what nature provided without man-made, artificial items filled with additives, preservatives, and toxins.

We enjoy wonderful lives in advanced cultures with modern amenities and manufacturing systems that produce economic bounties for businesses, their employees, and investors. However, the health of humankind diminishes in direct proportion to the distance from the natural, untouched, original food, water, and air God provided for us.

Convenience, speed, and greed typically make for poor health. To make a difference in your life, look for the healthiest options—not for what is quick, easy, cheap, and normal.

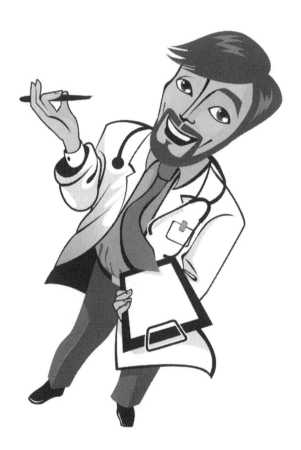

Chapter 8

HEALTHIEST OPTIONS

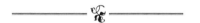

In diabetic terms, my body needed to be starved of carbohydrates. The brain needs carbohydrates to function, but just about everything we eat produces glucose, the primary carbohydrate that supports brain activity. My wife wants to lower her carbs in order to lose weight, but she gets dizzy and feels weak. Be watchful as you make changes.

Meats, poultry, fish, tofu, and eggs became the primary sources of protein, which were 60–70 percent of each of my two or three meals per day. I had one or two of them with a huge supply of fresh vegetables at each meal, including breakfast. It was weird, but it was also an awesome conversation starter.

Salad dressing with any carbs must be calculated into your twenty grams per day when you get started. I made my own salad dressing with organic apple cider vinegar (organic lemon juice works great too), extra virgin olive oil, crushed garlic, and a little sea salt for the most delicious and enjoyable carb-free salad dressing. Research the Paul Newman dressings to see which ones have very low carbs and meet your taste. This brand does not use any additives or preservatives, but the ingredients are not necessarily organic.

Do your best to buy organic, grass-fed, hormone-free meat and poultry. Be sure the fish is wild-caught and unprocessed. In other words, chicken nuggets and fish sticks are not to be considered. Dr. Al Sears, in one of his e-mail newsletters, explained how chemical additives on most processed foods, weaken the body in many unpredictable ways.[15] The weakest link in your body manifests itself as a diseased state—high blood pressure, gallstones, kidney malfunctions, immune disorders, and diabetes.

The Diabetes Reversal Report also recommends that diabetics avoid peanuts.[3] All other nuts are fine. Research different types of nuts to monitor your carbs. Cashews are relatively high in carbs; select nuts with the lowest carb content, especially when you get started with your twenty-grams-per-day regimen.

In addition, you must drink something. In this case, it is anything without sugar—even natural sugars, such as fruit juices and other drinks, and those with evaporated cane juice. Dairy products are definitely not recommended during this time (milk, cheese, cream cheese, yogurt, etc.). Your liquid of choice is lots of water. Select pure water; if possible, use alkaline water. The Budwig Center research indicates that taking steps to balance the pH toward alkaline levels seems to help restore health faster.[14]

Also, one Chinese remedy that really worked well consisted of wheat bran, whole-wheat flour, two eggs, and mixed vegetables. This was perhaps the most filling item. It was tasty and never caused a spike in blood sugar. I stumbled on this recipe on a website that claimed it would be effective in helping starve the body of carbs and restoring health to diabetics. Please see my version of this recipe in chapter 11 (Seriously Tasty and Filling Vegetable Sauté).

In addition to learning, have fun choosing the healthiest options through your own ongoing research.

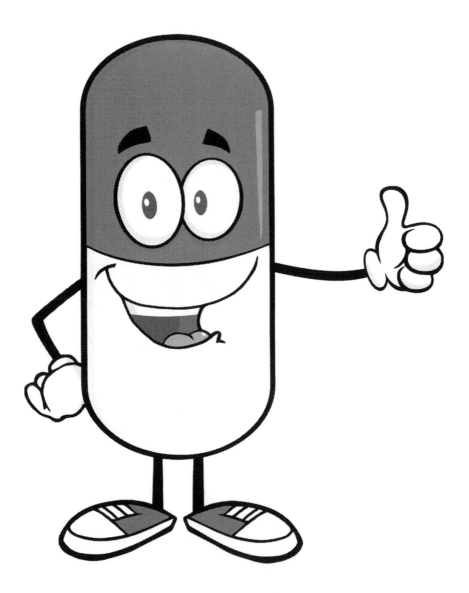

Chapter 9

NUTRITIONAL SUPPLEMENTS I TRIED (AND WHAT WORKED)

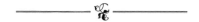

Below you will find a list of the supplements that I tried and the rationale behind each one. I researched in health food stores and websites, and used other materials along with my personal observations. This is from my personal research and experience, and it all may work much differently for you.

Item	Amount	Dosage /Research Findings / Personal Observations
Acetyl L-Carnitine	400–1000 mg	500 mg per day / nerve repair and cardiac tissue protection / enhanced brain clarity

Alpha Lipoic Acid[13]	<600 mg	200 mg per day / counters oxidative cell damage and reduces glucose in blood stream / glucose levels dropped significantly each time used
Calcium/Magnesium/ Vitamin D	500 mg / 250 mg / 200 IU	1 tablet per day / boosts beta cells in pancreas, reduces insulin resistance and replaces Mg lost due to insulin resistance / calmness even under pressure when taking this supplement
Choline	310 mg	1 capsule every other day / promotes healthy cell membranes / no observable effect
Chromium Picolinate	400 mcg	1 per day / improves cell membrane response to insulin / significant drop in blood sugar within 30–40 minutes after taking (prompted headaches if taken every day)

Cinnamon Organic[11,12]	500 mg	generally 2 tablets per meal (more if needed to bring sugar level down below 100 in 3–4 hours after a meal) made into a tea sometimes / lowers insulin resistance and cholesterol levels / easy to control blood sugar
Ginkgo Biloba	60 mg	1–2 per day / increases mental alertness, produces more pancreatic insulin, reduces chances of blood clots / with Ginkgo, I can give speeches more easily from memory and remember names more easily
StemEnhance	2 capsules	2 tablets per day / increases stem cells by 400 percent naturally / blood sugar patterns became smooth and normal after about thirty days

Glucoach from 4 Life, Inc.		took for one month and observed no effect on controlling blood sugar (it may have had long-term healing benefits, but I discontinued use after a short time)
Omega-3	1100 IU	1 capsule per day plus lots of salmon / prevents diabetic neuropathy, restores normal cardiac functions affected by diabetes, improves glucose control and weight loss / I was more energetic, had more endurance in a workday, and a lower heart rate
Pycnogenol	25 mg	2 tablets per day / capillary repair,especially eyes and extremities / fast restoration of clear eyesight—took me about two weeks for a noticeable difference

I discovered the real value of Alpha Lipoic Acid, which the body manufactures some on its own, from Sherry Rogers, MD, when she states that, "it should border on malpractice to forget to prescribe this nonprescription nutrient for diabetics" and goes on further to emphasize that, "it's a name you had better become familiar with if you are going to take charge and not only get yourself well, but keep yourself well."[13]

The United States Department of Agriculture research on cinnamon, published in July 2000, is also fascinating. I quote, "The search for a natural way to keep blood sugar levels normal began more than a decade ago when ARS chemist Richard A. Anderson and co-workers at the Beltsville (Maryland) Human Nutrition Research Center assayed plants and spices used in folk medicine. They found that a few spices—especially cinnamon—made fat cells much more responsive to insulin, the hormone that regulates sugar metabolism and thus controls the level of glucose in the blood."[11]

As you can see from the above, along with the many other recommended readings and websites listed in "A Bibliography with Useful Resources," there is quite a bit that one can do to learn about natural alternatives and practices to reverse diabetes.

One thing remains clear, and it is that with a few lifestyle changes to counter the many assaults on health found in our food, water, and environment, one can restore health fairly quickly—especially with type 2 diabetes.

Even with this encouraging research, however, it is imperative for you to monitor what each item does for you. Make note of your subjective observations and check your blood sugar levels in response to all items to chart the objective readings at each step and learn what really works for you. You and your doctor should work together to monitor and learn what these foods and supplements may be doing for you.

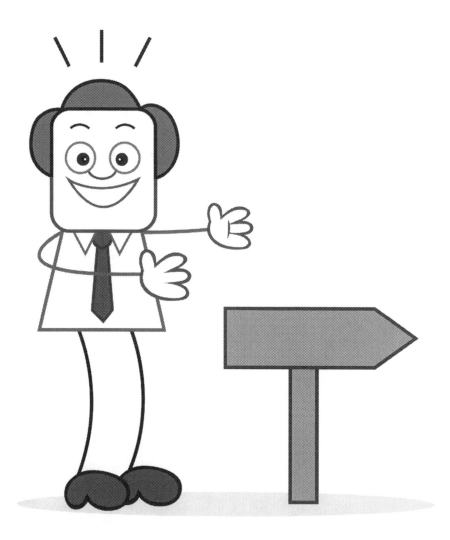

The information provided or referred to in this work – includes websites and their affiliates and sources -- is intended for your general knowledge only and is not a substitute for professional medical advice or treatment for specific medical conditions. You should not use this information to diagnose or treat a health problem or disease without consulting with a qualified healthcare provider. Please consult your healthcare provider with any questions or concerns you may have regarding your condition.

Chapter 10

MY STEP-BY-STEP REVIEW FOR SUCCESS

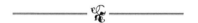

What should you do next? I can't prescribe for you, but here is what I did:

- Do the right thing. Be sure to check all options with your doctor.
- Verify that your body is producing insulin and that your problem is related to insulin resistance (type 2 diabetes).
- Make sure your doctor is aware of everything you are doing. Report any significant changes or concerns immediately.
- Take any medication that your doctor has prescribed according to the instructions.
- I started my research with a baseline. Make a recording table for your food and drink intake for two or three days before making any changes to diet or exercise. Record your blood sugar level to help you understand how your blood sugar level responds to your current lifestyle.

	Date	Baseline Data—Day 1 Nutritional Intake and Blood Glucose Levels							
		On Rising	Immediately before breakfast	30–45 minutes after breakfast	Immediately before lunch	30–45 minutes after lunch	Immediately before supper/dinner	30–45 minutes after supper/dinner	
Time									
Glucose									
Meal			Breakfast		Lunch		Dinner/Supper		
Intake Contains									

	Date	Baseline Data—Day 2 Nutritional Intake and Blood Glucose Levels							
		On Rising	Immediately before breakfast	30–45 minutes after breakfast	Immediately before lunch	30–45 minutes after lunch	Immediately before supper/dinner	30–45 minutes after supper/dinner	
Time									
Glucose									
Meal			Breakfast		Lunch		Dinner/Supper		
Intake Contains									

Date	Baseline Data—Day 3 Nutritional Intake and Blood Glucose Levels							
	On Rising	Immediately before breakfast	30–45 minutes after breakfast	Immediately before lunch	30–45 minutes after lunch	Immediately before supper/dinner	30–45 minutes after supper/dinner	
Time								
Glucose								
Meal		Breakfast		Lunch		Dinner/Supper		
Intake Contains								

Use your cell phone for cover when needed.

Practice taking your blood sugar readings immediately before and 30–45 minutes after each meal as well as first thing each morning before you make any changes to your diet or lifestyle. You will be taking your blood sugar on trains, on planes, at your desk, at work, and in restaurants. I learned to take my blood sugar in under one minute without being noticed—even during conference room meetings or on a plane. I tested it under tables and under my jacket. You can excuse yourself and use a restroom, being careful to clean your skin before and after. Practice a few times until you can do it without even looking and/or spreading out your paraphernalia. Just feel your way through the process, with a very occasional glance. When your glucometer beeps, look at your watch or cell phone to distract those around you.

Make the changes fun and educational.

While you are monitoring and recording your baseline data, you can continue researching and finalizing your meal and exercise plans. The most important thing is to make a decision about how much you will change and how quickly. Some of you will make numerous changes like I did immediately, and others will take one step at a time (a bit more methodical and incremental). Either one is fine.

The main thing is to identify the foods and beverages you will be using to reduce the carb intake to as close to twenty grams daily as you can. Use the websites listed later or any others you find to help you make food and beverage selections that make sense for you. This really makes it fun. Find foods you love or are willing to try that help you meet your health goals. The fun is in the process. Believe it can be done—and do not give up until you find it. The excitement is when you can shout, "I found it!"

Remember that meat, fish, eggs, chicken, tofu, TVP (textured vegetable protein, usually soy), and most fresh vegetables (natural, unprocessed, or raw) will be the main courses of all meals. Organics are preferred. Add raw nuts (except peanuts), selected beans, and grains (most grains are high in carbs, but in very small portions, they can be included) occasionally for variety. Avoid sugars, sweets, and pastries. Organic stevia worked well for me, and you can try other natural organic sweeteners with no glycemic value.

Make a list of your selected low-carb food items and their carbs per serving and glycemic value or load so you have a ready-made shopping list when you go. Make a combination of things you know you like and things you are willing to try. Add a few of the willing-to-try items until you find what you like.

Food / Beverage Item	Grams of Carbs / Serving Size		Net Carbs

As you practice using your own list to guide buying foods, eating, and combining them to make delicious meals, you will find it a lot easier to keep within your desired daily carb limits. I started with 20–25 grams of carbs per day.

After about six weeks, I missed my favorite rice, pasta, and potatoes. As I monitored my blood sugar, I found that I could increase my carb intake over the weekend and revert to my 20–25 daily grams during the week without disrupting my progress.

Use Internet power to make quick decisions.

Choose a website that helps you calculate the carbohydrate grams in each type of food by serving. The website that helped me make these decisions was http://www.carbs-information.com/carbs-in-food.htm.[2] By clicking on the type of food, it would take me to another window where I could specify a brand or a type, and it gave me the actual grams of carbohydrate per serving of that particular item. This is really great nutritional information to have for just general knowledge, but for the diabetic reversal, this is really a key step.

For example, if you select eggs, then poached eggs, and then eggs Benedict, you will find that the number of grams in eggs Benedict is much different. A two-egg Eggs Benedict serving has eighty grams of carbs, which would be way too many carbs. However, a poached or boiled egg has less than one gram of carbs. The site is a bit cumbersome since it has many helpful ads and definitions that require you to scroll each time you click to see the desired data on each item. In spite of that, I found it truly helpful.

Eat, drink, and monitor.

Once you have your foods selected and prepared, eat to your heart's content. Monitor your blood sugar with the same rigor as your first three days of baseline data. Remember that you are learning about your body and its response to foods you eat. Write notes about your food preparation so you can identify minor differences in glucose readings.

Check out the data. Do some of your own research into cinnamon, chromium picolinate, and other items I used to make a decision about where to start. Keep monitoring and learning. It is fascinating to see how your body responds. Use the results to determine if you need more or less of any of the items used to lower the readings.

Be methodical and consistent. Dr. Frank Yurasek has cured diabetes with acupuncture and dietary changes. He mentioned that I should eat at the same time every day and monitor the blood sugar at the same time every day. After learning what causes your blood sugar to spike sharply, modify your food intake and keep monitoring. I started monitoring seven times per day, and I went to two times per day after about four weeks. After just four weeks, I was able to see the downward trend of my blood sugar readings (particularly upon rising). Eating an early supper (no later than five thirty) made a huge difference.

Getting your fasting blood sugar below 100 mg/dl each morning is a milestone you want to see as the body retrains itself (see my chart for a twenty-one-day period after beginning to monitor twice per day). You will want to keep a table like the one on the previous page. If you can, make graph to see the trends of your blood sugar levels. Just watch for the milestones of lower blood glucose and try to understand what you did differently (whether it's a spike like mine on July 27 at six thirty in the morning or the really nice drop on July 31).

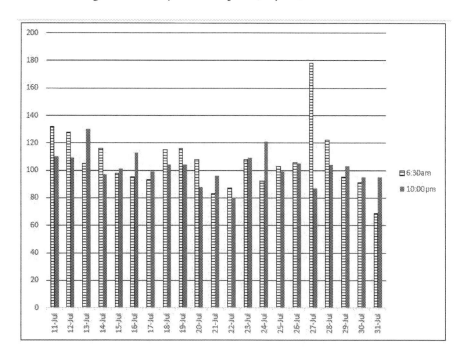

My spike was caused by eating a few cashews and almonds at two in the morning when I woke up hungry. It would have been better to eat a piece of fish or chicken—or not to have eaten at all. I should have filled up with water. After that spike, it took two days to come down below 100 mg/dl. To avoid being hungry in the middle of the night, I ate a little more at suppertime, which helped a lot for several months.

The nice drop on July 31 came from adding some cinnamon capsules during the day and evening to push the blood sugar down into the normal range.

This next step was for me a triumphant one. I trust that it will be the same for you. My body was responding to the regimen described above. My frequent urination was gone, and my body heat diminished (I used to be hot all the time). If I had some fruit, a sip of fruit juice, or even an extra spoon of rice or some raisins, I could feel my whole body pulsating, I realized that something was different about my body's response to food and beverages. I could see and feel my body changing as it adjusted to normal glucose levels. I decided to try one last supplement: StemEnhance from Stemtech. I wanted to be sure my cells were capable of responding favorably to the regimen before taking this leap. On September 1, I took the next step and pursued StemEnhance.

StemEnhance is made from algae known as *Aphanizomenon flos-aquae* that help the body produce its own stem cells.[4] When taken, the body has a higher concentration (400 percent higher) of new master cells available to replace the older, weaker cells. Stem cells naturally supply tissues where they are needed and can become any type of tissue. I added this item to the routine, and within twenty-one days, my blood sugar was consistently rising and falling at almost the normal cycle and range. My blood sugar would come down below 100 mg/dl within four hours of eating, and then later, it only took three hours to get to that level after eating.

To order StemEnhance, you must call StemTech. It is not sold in stores. A former pastor at my church told me of the research and suggested that I call someone who would know more about it. I found out that it is sold through independent distributors via direct sales, and I ordered it steadily for about six months. I firmly believe that God sent that pastor to our church for a short time just to share this information with me. He did other good things for our church, but I take this blessing personally.

You can get additional details on the Stemtech website (www.stemtechbiz.com) or at my exclusive health updates page—www.livingwelleveryday.com/updateme. The recommended dosage is one to two capsules twice per day, and it was about sixty dollars per month. Stemtech recently announced a new enhanced blend that allows the body to sustain higher levels of naturally produced stem cells for optimum health.

Two Essential Factors

There are two essential ingredients for turning around type 2 diabetes: a) modified food and liquid intake with restorative food supplements, and b) smart exercise to promote weight loss or muscle toning and reduce any excess of fat molecules from around the cell membranes. See how you can possibly do this in fast four-minute intervals.

Shake It Out in Four Minutes

High-intensity interval training (HIIT) is the best exercise for gaining or restoring health.[6] The physiological changes are significantly more accelerated, and the visible, measurable benefits of exercise are seen quickly. My friends (Jackie and Meredith) touted walking when I first discovered my diabetes. That is fine if you wish to control your condition. For those who can and wish to transform their bodies and establish normalcy of sugar regulation, I would, upon the approval of your physician, check out the following: P90X, Insanity, or Tabata. HIIT is based upon bursts of intense activity and short periods of rest. I used Tabata[5] and then graduated to Insanity. They are fun and extremely effective.

Tabata can be done at any time—even in church or business clothing. I used Tabata in my car one snowy night on a trip home from Detroit. My blood sugar had gone high (>180 mg/dl), and I had no more supplements with me. I knew I had to do something to continue training my body to stay in the range. I sat on the driver's side and went wild. I shook my arms in as many directions as I could and as vigorously as I could by using the Tabata principle, which means vigorous motion for twenty seconds and then resting for ten seconds. I repeated that seven times and completed the routine in four minutes. I shook my arms in the car that night, but, otherwise, did jumping jacks and leg lifts, and skipped rope. There are many videos and websites that describe this and similar exercise options adequately. The most thorough explanations I have found are located at the following websites:

- http://www.5min.com/Video/Tabata-Training-Method---Ep-32---Made-Fit-TV-87033743
- http://www.ncbi.nlm.nih.gov/pubmed/8897392? dopt=Abstract
- http://www.rosstraining.com/articles/tabataintervals.html

You can even download a Tabata clock that times your intervals according to your needs. The one I used is currently downloadable from www.beach-fitness.com/tabata.[7]

As a result of doing this routine in my car for eight minutes, my blood sugar dropped by thirty-two points in about thirty minutes. It was a thrilling victory!

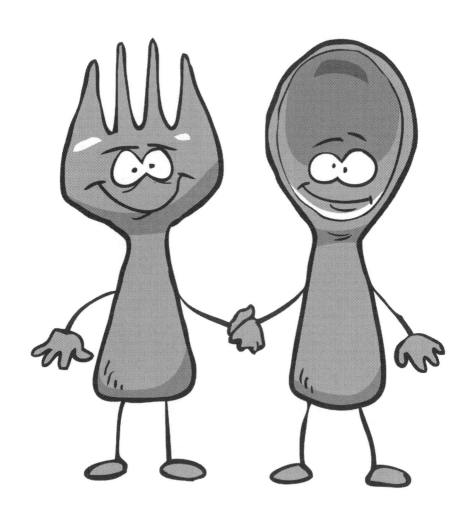

Chapter 11

DELICIOUS LOW-CARB RECIPES AND LITTLE-KNOWN NUTRITIONAL FACTS

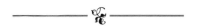

My most fascinating discovery was that I did not want to return to high-carb meals. The low-carb meals were so delicious and visually appealing. Restaurants will easily substitute vegetables or a larger salad in exchange for pasta or rice. Keep in mind that I used this strict format for only a few months. I now enjoy fruits, a piece of cake, or even some ice cream without seriously spiking my blood sugar levels. To get started, it's all low-carb. I tried my best to stay below twenty grams per day.

Keep in mind that 90 percent or more of my meals were organic vegetables, nuts, grains, seasonings, poultry, grass-fed beef, and wild-caught salmon. I researched and experimented with the following easy-to-make recipes to help retrain my body and provide them here to give you a wide variety of ideas for interesting and super delicious, low-carb recipes that you may wish to use right away.

Lightly Spiced Grilled Salmon
(4 Servings)

Spread a side of salmon with minced garlic, sprinkle with fresh basil, and layer sliced tomatoes on top. Put it on the grill (in foil) or in a lightly oiled saucepan medium to low heat. Do both sides for about 10 minutes until flaky and tender.

Ingredients

- 2 cloves garlic, minced
- 1 teaspoon sea salt, divided
- 1 tablespoon virgin coconut oil (better for diabetics and high heat)
- 1 wild-caught salmon fillet—whole
- 1/3 cup basil and an additional 1/4 cup thinly sliced fresh basil, divided
- 2 medium organic tomatoes, thinly sliced
- 1/4 teaspoon freshly ground black pepper

Directions

- Preheat grill or burner to medium.
- Mash minced garlic and 3/4 teaspoon sea salt on a cutting board with the flat side of the knife or a spoon until a paste forms. Transfer to a small bowl and stir in oil.
- Remove any bones as needed. Measure out a piece of heavy-duty foil (or use a double layer of regular foil) large enough for the wild-caught salmon fillet. Coat the foil with a little olive oil spray. Place the salmon skin-side down on the foil and spread the garlic mixture all over it. Sprinkle with 1/3 cup basil. Overlap tomato slices on top and sprinkle with the remaining 1/4 teaspoon salt and pepper.
- Transfer the salmon to the grill (with the foil) or saucepan. Grill or fry until the fish flakes easily, 10 to 12 minutes. Use two large

spatulas to slide the salmon from the foil or saucepan to a serving platter. Serve the salmon sprinkled with the remaining 1/4 cup basil.

During the initial few weeks, as I retrained my body, I stayed away from all of these foods:

wheat, wheat-based products	bread crumbs, croutons
breads—all types (1/2 slice per day max)	milk, yogurt, all cheeses
potatoes—all types	fruit
canned soups	all cereals and granolas
chips and pretzels	barley, oats, millet, etc.
beans (except kidney/ black soy)	okra
barbecued meats and poultry	mayonnaise
frozen meals	deli meats with any additives
carbonated beverages	roasted vegetables
all roasted/deep-fried foods	butter and margarine

Some of the above foods may surprise you, but others are obviously high in carbs. Advanced Glycation End products (AGEs) are often overlooked in food selection and food preparation for diabetics.[8,9] In general, the higher the heat used to prepare foods—such as barbecue, roasting, and other dry-heat methods—the higher the harmful content of AGEs we consume. This is especially true with fats, meats, and meat substitutes, but it also applies to things like corn.

Fascinating research found in the National Library of Medicine and the National Institutes of Health indicates that AGEs can affect cellular sensitivity to insulin, causing symptoms of diabetes and other diseases:

http://www.ncbi.nlm.nih.gov/pubmed/15281050
http://www.ncbi.nlm.nih.gov/pmc/articles/PMC3704564/

For this reason, many of these recipes recommend low to medium heat whenever needed.

See these and more of Dale's low-carb recipes online at www. livingwelleveryday.com/recipes-diabetes4/

Seriously Tasty and Filling Vegetable Sauté

As I was researching various cultures and diets for curing diabetes, I found this tasty, filling recipe that I adopted and modified using other nutritional data, from Chinese Natural Cures written by Henry C Lu.[10] The article said it is used in China. I ended up bringing it on planes so I would have some for every meal!

Add a handful of each item to a saucepan with virgin coconut oil, and sauté on low to medium heat until very slightly cooked:

- florets of organic broccoli
- organic cauliflower
- organic shredded or diced carrots
- organic cabbage and any other organic vegetable you have on hand

Turn fire very low while preparing for the next step—or remove from fire completely.

Add a mixture of:

- 60 percent wheat bran (fiber)
- 40 percent organic wheat flour (example 1 cup flour and 1 1/2 cups wheat bran)

Make a hole in the middle of your mixture in the saucepan to add 1–2 eggs and 1/2 cup alkaline water. Keep water on hand to moisten as needed. Return fire to medium heat and stir mixture until deep brown. Add a little water, as needed, to keep slightly moist while mixing.

Sprinkle sea salt, chili pepper, oregano, basil, or any of your favorite seasonings to taste and enjoy. It's delicious! Post your comments on my blog at http://livingwelleveryday.com/recipes-diabetes

The research from a controlled China study in 1989 by Zhonghua Nei Ke Za Zhi identified that wheat bran lowered blood glucose and enhanced the intestinal absorption of zinc (an essential mineral for blood sugar control).[17]

Filling Lunch Salad

Ingredients

- 1 cup shredded cabbage—purple or green
- 1 cup chopped kale (lettuce can be substituted)
- 2 slices tomato
- 3–5 slices cucumber
- 1 chopped scallion
- 1 organic chicken (cut or broken into small pieces)
- 2–3 teaspoons virgin cold pressed olive oil
- 1½ teaspoons apple cider vinegar
- sea salt and pepper to taste

When cooking chicken during this early phase, use a poaching method to prepare. I learned this from Chef Darin at www.chefdarin.com ("Why Boiled Chicken Is Bad").[16] For those who must have very rich seasoning, this method works without all the AGEs from the oven, saucepan, or grill. Poaching is essentially bringing water to a boil with all the seasonings you want to be in the chicken, removing it from the heat, and placing the chicken in the seasoned water to cook without boiling. This makes great, melt-in-your-mouth chicken for any purpose.

One of the reasons why salads like these are great is due to the low carb count and the high mineral content, especially copper, zinc, magnesium, and calcium.

See these and more of Dale's low-carb recipes online at www.livingwelleveryday.com/recipes-diabetes4/

Soaked Whole Grain and Seed Recipe

Whole grains are highly recommended for diabetics. Ray Sahelian, MD, states:

> Those who eat the whole grains have a lower risk of heart disease, stroke, and diabetes, not to mention better colon health. The reasons for the health benefits aren't hard to fathom. Whole grains include not just the starchy interior of a kernel, but also the fibrous bran that surrounds it, together with the vitamin- and mineral-rich germ (or seed). In contrast, fluffy white refined flour—the kind in most cakes, cookies, and crackers—has the highly nutritious bran and germ stripped away.[18]

In 1977, Curtis Golden, ND, taught me how to gain the optimum benefit from whole grains. This recipe retains almost all the nutrients in the grains in an easy-to-prepare format. All the ingredients must be seeds or grains that have not been irradiated or processed in any way - capable of germination or sprouting.

The whole-grain and seed recipe provided the nutrients so my hair that fell out from the right side of my head—as I mentioned earlier—started growing back in about two weeks.

Ingredients

- 1 tablespoon barley seeds
- 2 tablespoons oats
- 2 tablespoons millet
- 1 tablespoon buckwheat
- 1 tablespoon wheat berries
- 2 tablespoons chia seeds
- 2 tablespoons flaxseeds
- 2 tablespoons quinoa (not in Dr. Golden's original recipe)

- distilled water
- organic stevia or other natural sweetener with zero carbs (optional)

Quinoa, like other grains, is incredibly anti-inflammatory and addresses obesity, diabetes, and cardiovascular diseases. It also provides high levels of protein and magnesium. Magnesium is an ideal mineral for most diabetics.

- Mix the dry seeds and grains, and place in a stainless-steel or ceramic bowl.
- Add distilled water to a level about 1/2 inch to 3/4 inch above the top of the mixture.
- Place in refrigerator for 24–48 hours to soak (releases a host of therapeutic enzymes while the seeds germinate relatively slowly under refrigeration).
- Keep refrigerated until totally consumed.

Eat 1–2 tablespoons twice per day with a dash of optional stevia as a sweetener just before eating. This preparation can also be used as a topping on vegetable salads. If you find it hard to chew, place the soaked mixture in a blender or emulsifier with distilled water or cinnamon tea and drink immediately. I found that with cinnamon tea, my blood sugar would go a little low. I found it best to check my blood sugar about thirty minutes after consuming the tea to avoid a level that was too low.

After my body began returning to normal, I started adding dried fruit to the mixture and soaking them along with the whole grains. As with all other foods, I try to find organic or pesticide-free versions of dried fruit.

Bean and Kale Bonanza

Ingredients

- 2–3 tablespoons olive oil
- 4 medium garlic cloves
- 4 cups organic kale,* chopped
- 1/4 cup uncooked organic cannellini beans* (cook 2 cups or more in boiling water—approximately 35 minutes—to store in the refrigerator for additional servings at a later time)
- 1/8 teaspoon black pepper
- 1/8 teaspoon sea salt (if needed)
- 1/2 cup chicken broth (If available, use low sodium Vegebase chicken broth powder from Vogue Cuisine. This organic brand has no preservatives or additives. It is gluten-free and a great salt substitute with exquisite broth flavor.)

Directions

- Add and spread oil in a skillet. Set over medium heat, add garlic, and cook until golden and slightly softened. Add kale and toss to coat. Reduce heat slightly and cook about 3 minutes, or until wilted—depends on type of kale.
- Add cooked beans, season with salt and pepper, and toss gently. Add broth, reduce heat to low, and cook about 10 minutes (or until beans have soaked up the flavor and kale is flaccid).

*I also substituted organic pinto beans, mung beans, soybeans, black-eyed peas (limit amount—high in carbs), and others. Check the carb counter to see which ones have low carbs. I also substituted other green leafy vegetables, such as spinach, collard greens, callaloo, and bok choy. I even mixed them all together.

Ethnic Salted Codfish and Cabbage
(4–6 servings)

Ingredients

- 1/2 pound salted boneless codfish (found in Caribbean or Hispanic stores) (Spanish: *bacalao sin hueso*)
- 1 medium head of organic cabbage, shredded (red or green or ½ red and ½ green cabbage for variety
- 1 large organic onion (purple or yellow), diced
- 1 clove garlic, minced
- 3 tablespoons virgin organic coconut oil
- 1/2 teaspoon black pepper (can use 1/4 teaspoon of cayenne red pepper)

Directions

- Soak the salted codfish in distilled water overnight (about 6–7 hours to remove excess salt, soak longer if on a low-salt diet).
- Tear or cut fish into small to medium-sized pieces.
- Sauté onions and garlic in oil on medium heat in a skillet.
- Add fish and sauté for another 2 minutes on medium to low heat until slightly soft or golden.
- Add cabbage with some pepper to taste.
- Stir until soft and a little juicy.
- Serve piping hot and enjoy this almost zero-carb meal.

Chicken Casserole with Broccoli Garnish

Ingredients

- 3 large organic chicken breasts
- 2 cups organic broccoli
- 1 organic onion, chopped
- 2 cups fresh mushrooms, sliced
- 1 cup no-chicken broth (Vogue Cuisine Vegebase preferred)
- 1 cup distilled or alkaline water
- 2 garlic cloves, chopped
- 1–2 cup(s) nutritional yeast flakes or powder (cheese substitute)
- Sea salt and pepper

Directions

- Cook and season chicken with salt and pepper. Poach (if just starting this regimen to avoid AGEs). Otherwise, bake, steam, or fry. Chop or shred and set aside.
- Cook broccoli spears or florets. Steam or boil (no need to season).
- Sauté onion and garlic just until slightly soft (2–3 minutes).
- Mix broth and water.
- In a 13 x 9–inch pan, layer the chopped or shredded chicken on the bottom, followed by broccoli, onion and garlic, mushrooms, broth mixture, salt, and pepper on top.
- Bake at 350°F for 30 minutes.
- Sprinkle nutritional yeast evenly over the top.

Barley Lentil Soup

Ingredients

- olive oil cooking spray
- 1 cup sliced organic onion
- 1 teaspoon minced organic garlic
- 1 cup organic carrots, sliced
- 1 cup organic celery, sliced
- 15-ounce can stewed diced organic tomatoes
- 3 cups Vogue Cuisine Vegebase broth
- 3 cups water
- 1 cup dry organic lentils, rinsed
- 1/2 cup golden organic barley, whole grain
- 1/2 teaspoon dried thyme
- 1 teaspoon dried oregano
- 1 teaspoon dried basil
- 1/4 teaspoon black pepper, to taste

Directions

- Spray a large saucepan with cooking spray, and heat over medium.
- Sauté the garlic and onion until golden brown (about 1 or 2 minutes).
- Add the rest of the ingredients, and bring to a boil. Reduce the heat so the mixture is at a light simmer. Cover and cook until the barley and lentils are tender (about 1 hour to 1 1/2 hours). Serve hot.
- Great protein and highly complex carbs. Serve with a salad, or enjoy as is.

Easy Split Pea Soup

Ingredients

- 1 cup organic onion, chopped
- 1 cup organic carrot, chopped
- 1 cup organic kale, chopped
- 1 clove organic garlic, minced
- 3 organic celery stalks, chopped
- 12 ounces dry organic split peas
- 3 cups vegetable broth made from Vogue Cuisine Vegebase
- 2 cups distilled or alkaline water
- 1 bay leaf
- 1 teaspoon dried thyme
- 1 teaspoon dried oregano
- 1/4 teaspoon black pepper

Directions

- Place all ingredients in a large pot. Bring to a boil, and then reduce heat to simmer.
- Cook covered, until the peas are tender. Remove cover to increase evaporation for an additional 10 minutes. Serve hot.

Eggplant Burgers

Ingredients

- 1 medium eggplant
- ¼ cup alkaline water
- 1 tablespoon virgin coconut oil
- 1/2 cup nutritional yeast
- 10 large pieces organic lettuce leaves
- 2 organic tomatoes, medium

Directions

- Peel eggplant and cut crosswise into 10 or more slices (1/4-inch thick).
- Place the eggplant slices and cook in a saucepan for about 10 minutes or until slightly cooked.
- Drain off any excess water.
- Melt coconut oil in a large skillet over medium heat. Sauté eggplant slices until lightly toasted on each side.
- Sprinkle nutritional yeast onto each eggplant slice, and when completely moist, remove from the skillet.
- Place eggplant on a lettuce leaf and tomato slices.
- Add seasoning or toppings according to taste.
- Wrap eggplant in the lettuce leaf for a delicious treat.

See these and more of Dale's low-carb recipes online at www.livingwelleveryday.com/recipes-diabetes4/

Grilled Salmon Pepper Steaks

This recipe works best with overnight marinating.

Ingredients

- 2 tablespoons black pepper
- 2 pounds wild Alaskan or Washington salmon, fresh
- 2/3 cup white rice vinegar
- 2 tablespoons lemon juice
- 2 tablespoons Dijon mustard
- 1 tablespoon sesame oil
- 1/4 teaspoon salt
- 4 garlic cloves
- 1/4 teaspoon cornstarch

Directions

- Rinse fish; pat dry with paper towels. Cut into 4–6 pieces, approximately 5 ounces each, if necessary.
- Sprinkle salt evenly over the fish. Sprinkle black pepper (freshly cracked works best) evenly over both sides of each piece of salmon, and place in a 13 x 9–inch baking dish lightly coated with cooking spray.
- Combine vinegar, lemon juice, mustard, sesame oil, salt, and garlic (peeled and minced) in a small bowl; stir well. Pour vinegar mixture over fish.
- Cover and marinate for 1 hour, turning fish occasionally.
- Prepare grill. Remove fish from dish, reserving marinade. Place fish on grill rack lightly coated with oil, and grill 5 minutes on each side, basting frequently with half of the reserved marinade.
- Combine remaining half of marinade and cornstarch in a small saucepan; bring to a boil and cook 1 minute or until thickened, stirring constantly with a wire whisk.
- To serve, spoon about 1 tablespoon of sauce over each piece of fish. Serve with steamed broccoli or other vegetables, if desired.

Meatloaf with Tomato Sauce

Ingredients

- 3 organic/free-range eggs
- 1 slice organic bread, whole-wheat without preservatives
- 4 fluid ounces organic almond milk
- 2 tablespoons nutritional yeast
- 2 teaspoons parsley, dried
- 1/8 teaspoon black pepper
- 2 organic garlic cloves
- 12 ounces organic/grass-fed beef, sirloin, ground, extra lean
- 8 ounces organic sausage turkey, Italian (Italian Sausage Tofurky can also be used)
- 1/2 cup organic spaghetti sauce

Directions

- Preheat oven to 375°F.
- In a large bowl, combine eggs, bread (cut or torn into small pieces), milk, nutritional yeast, parsley, pepper, and garlic (peeled and minced).
- Add ground beef and sausage (casings removed); mix thoroughly. Shape meat mixture into a round loaf (9 inches in diameter).
- Place loaf on the unheated rack of a broiler pan or a roasting pan with a rack. Spread spaghetti sauce evenly over top.
- Bake for 25–30 minutes or until a thermometer inserted into the middle of the loaf registers 160°F and juices run clear.
- Transfer to a serving platter; sprinkle with herbs of choice, such as basil, thyme, or garlic powder. Cut into wedges to serve.
- Serve with a tossed salad and hot cooked orzo or risotto, if desired.

Stuffed Peppers with Black Beans and Quinoa

Ingredients

- 1 tablespoon oil (extra-virgin olive, canola, or grape-seed oil)
- 1 medium onion, diced
- 2 medium carrots, diced or grated
- 2 cloves garlic, minced
- 3/4 cup quinoa, dry (follow rinsing directions if on package)
- 3/4 teaspoon sea salt
- 3 large organic peppers, bell (any color)
- 2 cups cooked organic beans, black, no salt added, drained after cooking
- 6 ounces tomato sauce, no added salt
- 1 teaspoon chili powder
- 3/4 teaspoon cumin, ground
- 1/2 teaspoon paprika, smoked (may substitute regular paprika)
- 1/2 teaspoon oregano, dried
- 2 tablespoon cilantro, fresh, chopped (optional)
- 3/4 cup nutritional yeast flakes

Directions

- Preheat the oven to 375°F. Line a rimmed baking sheet with aluminum foil.
- Heat the olive oil in a 3-quart saucepan over medium heat. Add the onion and carrot, and sauté until the vegetables have softened (about 8 minutes). Add the garlic, and sauté for 2 minutes, stirring frequently. Add the quinoa, 1 1/2 cups water, and the salt. Bring the water to a boil, and then reduce the heat to low, cover the saucepan, and simmer for 20 to 25 minutes, or until all of the liquid has been absorbed.
- While the quinoa is cooking, prepare the peppers. Cut the peppers in half lengthwise, trim the stems, and scoop out all seeds and membranes. Arrange the peppers cut-side up on the

baking sheet, and mist the peppers liberally with oil spray. Bake for 15 minutes to soften the peppers. Remove from oven.

- Add the black beans, tomato sauce, chili powder, cumin, paprika, and oregano to the quinoa, and mix thoroughly. Stir in the cilantro, if using. Divide the quinoa mixture evenly between the six pepper halves and pat the filling down to pack it into the pepper cups. Bake the stuffed peppers for 25 minutes. Top the peppers with the nutritional yeast (cheese substitute) during the last 5 minutes of baking -- if desired.

See these and more of Dale's low-carb recipes online at www.livingwelleveryday.com/recipes-diabetes4/

Roasted Vegetables with Rosemary

Ingredients

- 2 tomatoes, large, chopped
- 2 carrots, thinly sliced
- 1 zucchini, thinly sliced
- 1 pepper, red, bell, chopped
- 1 cup broccoli florets, small
- 1 onion, red, thinly sliced
- 1/2 cup corn (frozen, thawed, or fresh kernels)
- 2 tablespoon coconut oil
- 1/4 cup fresh rosemary, minced
- 1/4 teaspoon red pepper flakes
- 1/4 teaspoon sea salt
- 1/4 cup organic balsamic vinegar
- 2 cloves organic garlic, minced

Directions

- Preheat the oven to 400°F. Line a baking sheet with aluminum foil or parchment paper.
- In a large bowl, combine the tomatoes, carrots, zucchini, bell pepper, broccoli, onion, and corn.
- Add the coconut oil, and rub it over all the vegetables until well coated.
- Add the rosemary, vinegar, garlic, red pepper flakes, and sea salt. Mix well.
- Spread out evenly on the prepared baking sheet.
- Sprinkle with 3–5 tablespoons of water.
- Roast for 20–25 minutes, turning occasionally, until the vegetables are tender and the tomatoes begin to fall apart.
- Serve immediately.

Healthy Kale Snack

Ingredients

- 1 bunch organic kale, large
- olive oil spray (organic from Trader Joe's)
- nutritional yeast (for cheesy flavor)
- sea salt

Directions

- Preheat the oven to 375°F. Coat two large baking sheets with oil spray (chips will be crispiest if baked directly on the baking sheet, without aluminum foil).
- Trim the stem ends off the kale, and cut or tear the leaves into 2-inch pieces (some stores sell chopped organic kale).
- Divide the kale pieces between the two baking sheets, and spread them into a single, even layer.
- Liberally mist the kale with organic olive oil spray, and lightly sprinkle with salt and nutritional yeast.
- Bake for 8–10 minutes, or until the kale is crispy to the touch and the edges are beginning to brown.

Tofu, Cauliflower, and Chickpea Curry

Ingredients

- 1 tablespoon virgin coconut oil or grape-seed oil
- 1 1/2 teaspoon mustard seed, whole
- 1 teaspoon cumin seeds, whole
- 1 large onion, diced
- 4 cloves organic garlic, minced
- 1 tablespoon fresh ginger root, minced
- 4 teaspoons Madras curry powder or paste
- 1 teaspoon turmeric
- 1/4 teaspoon cumin
- 1/8 teaspoon cayenne or hot chili pepper
- 1 head organic cauliflower, cut into bite-sized florets
- 1 package organic tofu, extra firm, drained and pressed to remove excess water, and cut into 1/4-inch cubes
- 1 can organic tomatoes, diced
- 1/4 cup broth (made from Vogue Cuisine Vegebase powder or water)
- 1 can organic garbanzo beans (chickpeas), drained and rinsed
- 1 teaspoon sea salt
- 1 whole fresh organic lemon with rind, juice
- 1/4 cup cilantro

Directions

- Heat the oil in a large pot or deep skillet over medium-high heat. Add the mustard and cumin seeds, and cook until they begin to pop (about 1 minute).
- Reduce the heat to medium. Add the onion and cook until translucent and soft (6–8 minutes). Add the garlic, ginger, curry powder or paste, and cayenne, and cook for 1 minute, stirring constantly.

- Add the cauliflower florets, cubed tofu, canned tomatoes (with liquids), and broth or water, and stir well. Bring the liquid to a boil. Reduce the heat to medium-low, cover the pot, and simmer for 15 minutes, or until the cauliflower is nearly tender. Add the chickpeas. Season with salt, and simmer uncovered for 10 minutes.
- Stir in the lemon juice. Serve the curry alone or over a bed of hot cooked organic brown rice (regular or brown basmati). Garnish with cilantro, if using.

EPILOGUE

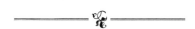

I sincerely hope you can feel my excitement and passionate desire to share this information with you. My family doctor, Dr. Amin, has encouraged me to write this book because of the stats shown below. He has said on more than one occasion that he would love to share this story with his other diabetic patients.

Item	Reading on July 23, 2009	Reading on December 30, 2010
A1C	12.1	5.7
Cholesterol total	184	132
Triglycerides	389	88
CHOL/HDLC Ratio	5.4	2.6
Glucose-fasting	398	98

I hope your journey will be even more dramatic than mine. Do the research, practice healthy living as your own body dictates, make it a skill that you can share with others, and love the one life you have so you can give glory to God. Praise Him! Praise Him! Praise Him!

Never miss an update from Dale. Join Dale's exclusive *Diabetes Annihilated Naturally Group* on Facebook at www.facebook.com/groups/dalecampbell/ using published research, reports, recipes, and more, to optimize health, help annihilate diabetes and inform healthy life-style choices that make a difference for his readers.

A Bibliography with Useful Resources

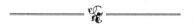

1. "Carb Counter Website," accessed 3/31/2015 http://www.carb-counter.org/.
2. "Carbohydrates in Food," accessed 8/12/2009 http://www.carbs-information.com/carbs-in-food.htm.
3. Barton, Joe, "Diabetes Reversal Report" accessed 7/3/2009 http://diabetesreversed.com/index5.php.
4. "Stemtech website" accessed 8/17/2010 www.stemtechbiz.com.
5. Tabata, I., Nishimura, K., Kouzaki, M., Hirai, Y., Ogita, F., Miyachi, M., Yamamoto, K. "Effects of moderate-intensity endurance and high-intensity intermittent training on anaerobic capacity and VO2max." Med Sci Sports Exerc. 1996 Oct;28(10):1327-30, accessed 11/22/2009 http://www.ncbi.nlm.nih.gov/pubmed/8897392.
6. "HIIT Training: The Cure for Insulin Resistance, Type 2 Diabetes, metabolic Disease and Obesity?," accessed 1/10/2010 http://healthhabits.ca/2009/01/28/hiit-training-the-cure-for-insulin-resistance-type-2-diabetes-metabolic-disease-and-obesity/.
7. "Tabata timer" accessed 12/4/2010 www.beach-fitness.com/tabata/.

8. Goldberg T, Cai W, Peppa M, Dardaine V, Baliga BS, Uribarri J, Vlassara H. "Advanced Glycation End Products in commonly consumed foods," J Am Diet Assoc. 2005 Apr;105(4): 647, accessed 01/02/2010 http://www.ncbi.nlm.nih.gov/pubmed/15281050.

9. Vlassara H, Uribarri J, "Advanced glycation end products (AGE) and diabetes: cause, effect, or both?," Curr Diab Rep. 2014 Jan;14(1):453. doi: 10.1007/s11892-013-0453-1, accessed 3/03/2014 http://www.ncbi.nlm.nih.gov/pubmed/24292971.

10. Lu, Henry C. "Chinese Natural Cures" accessed 3/18/15 https://books.google.com/books?id=3biQHyIKOBcC&pg=PA469&lpg=PA469&dq=chinese+wheat+bran+mixed+with+vegetables+diabetes&source=bl&ots=qGxGup2xS2&sig=u7Qz2r-toOLc_k8ibW_6vNuoDmzU&hl=en&sa=X&ei=wcsJVZ-PlMfPIsQStroGQAQ&ved=0CEsQ6AEwBw#v=onepage&q=chinese%20wheat%20bran%20mixed%20with%20vegetables%20diabetes&f=false.

11. McBride, Judy "Cinnamon Extracts Boost Insulin Sensitivity," *Agricultural Research Magazine*, July 2000. http://agresearchmag.ars.usda.gov/2000/jul/cinn/.

12. Khan A, Safdar M, Ali Khan MM, Khattak KN, Anderson RA, "Cinnamon improves glucose and lipids of people with type 2 diabetes," Diabetes Care. 2003 Dec 26 (12): 3215-8, accessed 12/14/2009 http://www.ncbi.nlm.nih.gov/pubmed/14633804.

13. Rogers, Sherry A. MD, Detoxify or Die (New York: Prestige Publishing, 2002), 74, 89-91.

14. "pH Balancing is a Must to Regain Your Health," last accessed 3/18/2015 http://www.budwigcenter.com/acid-ph-dangers/#.VRysRPnF9PM.

15. Sears, Al MD, "Spicy Secret to Safe Blood Sugar," accessed 11/06/2013, http://alsearsmd.benchmarkmails26.com/c/l?u=2EBF9DA&e=3D4281&c=3E39A&t=0&l=C1B413&email=kB4lCkdXRiUWiMOFunNoXDciHg%2FVbFy1.

16. Sehnert, Chef Darin, "Why Boiled Chicken Is Bad?," accessed 8/9/2013, http://www.chefdarin.com/2011/04/why-boiled-chicken-is-bad/.

17. Liu ZQ, Chao CS, Wu HW, "Investigation of the effect of a diet with wheat bran on the metabolic balances of Zn, Cu, Ca and Mg in diabetics" Zhonghua Nei Ke Za Zhi. 1989 Dec;28(12):741-4, 769, accessed 3/22/2010 http://www.ncbi.nlm.nih.gov/pubmed/2561477.

18. Sahelian, Ray, MD, "Whole Grains and Cereal Health Benefit" last modified 01/06/2015 www.raysahelian.com/wholegrains.html.

Printed in the United States
By Bookmasters